Obesity is Big Issue, Be Safe By Knowing About Obesity

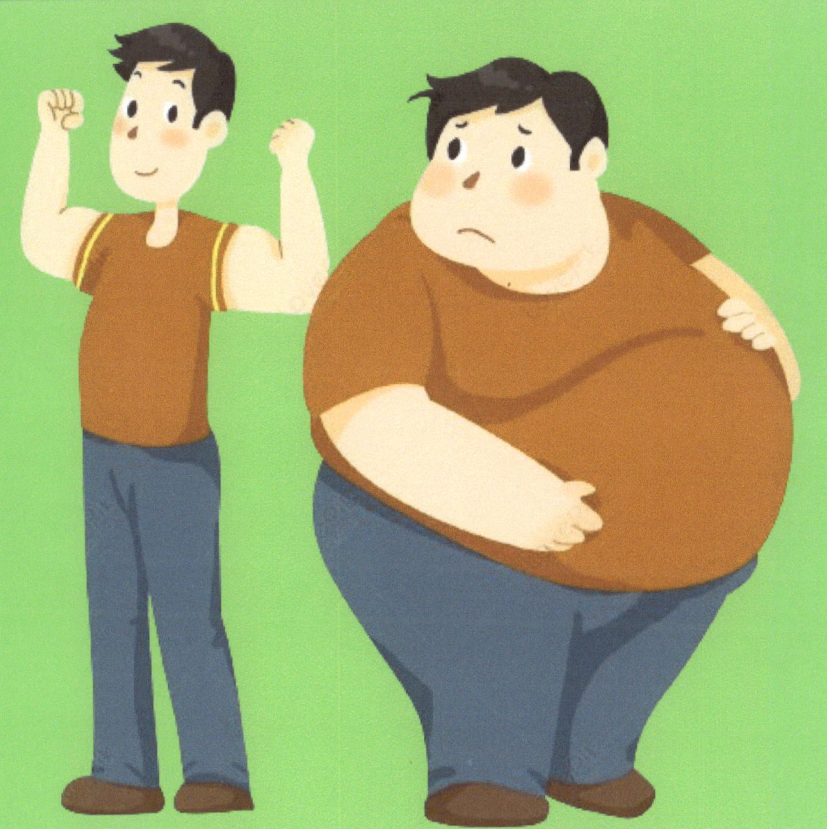

"Obesity is the silent killer that creeps into our lives, causing devastating health problems over time."

About the Authors

MR. JAYAPRATHAP NAGARAJ

Mr. Jayaprathap Nagaraj has a diverse background in both the fields of pharmacy and sports science. He holds a Bachelor of Pharmacy degree and has furthered his expertise with a Sports Degree from the prestigious National Institute of Sports. With a profound understanding of pharmaceuticals and a strong foundation in sports science, Mr. Jayaprathap Nagaraj brings a unique perspective to the topic of obesity management. His interdisciplinary approach combines medication knowledge with practical insights into physical activity, making him a valuable contributor to this comprehensive guide.

DR. SUVATHI VASAN

Dr. Suvathi Vasan is currently in the final year (2024) of her Bachelor of Naturopathy and Yogic Sciences (BNYS) at the Government Yoga and Naturopathy Medical College. Her deep understanding of natural and holistic healing practices, along with her commitment to integrative health, positions her as an authority on the subjects of naturopathy and yoga.

Dr. Suvathi Vasan's academic and practical experiences enable her to provide readers with effective, natural approaches to managing and reducing obesity. Her contributions emphasize the importance of holistic care in achieving long-term health and wellness.

MR. ABINESH KUMAR EPN

Mr. Abinesh Kumar EPN has completed his Bachelor of Exercise Physiology and Nutrition, equipping him with in-depth knowledge of how exercise and diet impact the human body. His expertise lies in understanding the intricate balance between physical activity and nutrition, essential components in the fight against obesity. Mr. Kumar's scientific approach to exercise physiology and his detailed understanding of nutritional needs provide practical and evidence-based strategies for weight management. His insights help readers develop effective, sustainable diet and exercise plans tailored to their specific needs.

Together, Mr. Jayaprathap Nagaraj, Dr. Suvathi Vasan, and Mr. Abinesh Kumar EPN offer a comprehensive and multidisciplinary approach to understanding and managing obesity.

Their combined expertise spans the fields of pharmacy, sports science, naturopathy, yoga, exercise physiology, and nutrition, ensuring a holistic and informed perspective on the complexities of obesity and its management. This book serves as a valuable resource for anyone seeking to understand obesity, its causes, and effective strategies for recovery through diet, naturopathy, yoga, and exercise.

Authors

MR.Jayaprathap Nagaraj, Nis, B.Pharm,

Dr.Suvathi vasan, BNYS

MR.Abinesh Kumar Nagaraj, EPN

A Motivational Message from the Authors

EMBRACE THE JOURNEY TO HEALTH AND WELLNESS

Dear Reader,

Embarking on the journey to health and wellness is a powerful decision that can transform your life. As experts in pharmacy, sports science, naturopathy, yoga, exercise physiology, and nutrition, we are here to support and inspire you every step of the way.

Mr. Jayaprathap Nagaraj:

As someone who has combined the disciplines of pharmacy and sports science, I understand the importance of a holistic approach to health. Remember, every small step you take towards better health is a victory. Embrace the power of movement and the benefits of an active lifestyle. Your body is capable of incredible things, and with the right mindset, you can achieve your goals.

Dr. Suvathi Vasan:

In my journey through naturopathy and yoga, I've seen firsthand the transformative effects of natural healing and mindful practices.

Your body has an amazing ability to heal and rejuvenate itself. By incorporating naturopathy and yoga into your routine, you can find balance, reduce stress, and foster a deeper connection with your body. Believe in your inner strength and the power of holistic care to guide you on this path.

Mr. Abinesh Kumar EPN:

With my background in exercise physiology and nutrition, I can assure you that understanding and nurturing your body through proper nutrition and physical activity is key to achieving lasting health. Focus on nourishing your body with wholesome foods and embracing regular exercise as a joyful part of your life. Each healthy choice you make brings you closer to a fitter, stronger, and more vibrant you.

Remember, the journey to reducing obesity and improving your health is not a sprint but a marathon. It requires patience, dedication, and self-compassion. Celebrate your progress, no matter how small, and stay committed to your goals. You have the power to make positive changes and create a healthier, happier life for yourself.

Believe in yourself and trust in the process. We believe in you, and we are here to support you every step of the way. Let's embark on this journey together and achieve the vibrant health and wellness you deserve.

With motivation and support,

Mr. Jayaprathap Nagaraj,
Dr. Suvathi Vasan, and
Mr. Abinesh Kumar EPN

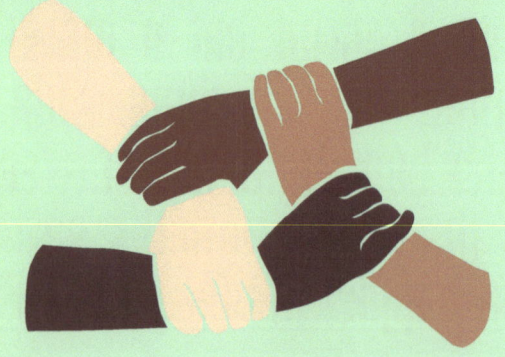

OBESITY

What is Obesity?

Definition

Obesity is a medical condition characterized by an excessive accumulation of body fat that presents a risk to health. It is typically measured using the Body Mass Index (BMI), a calculation based on height and weight: A BMI of 30 or higher is classified as obese:

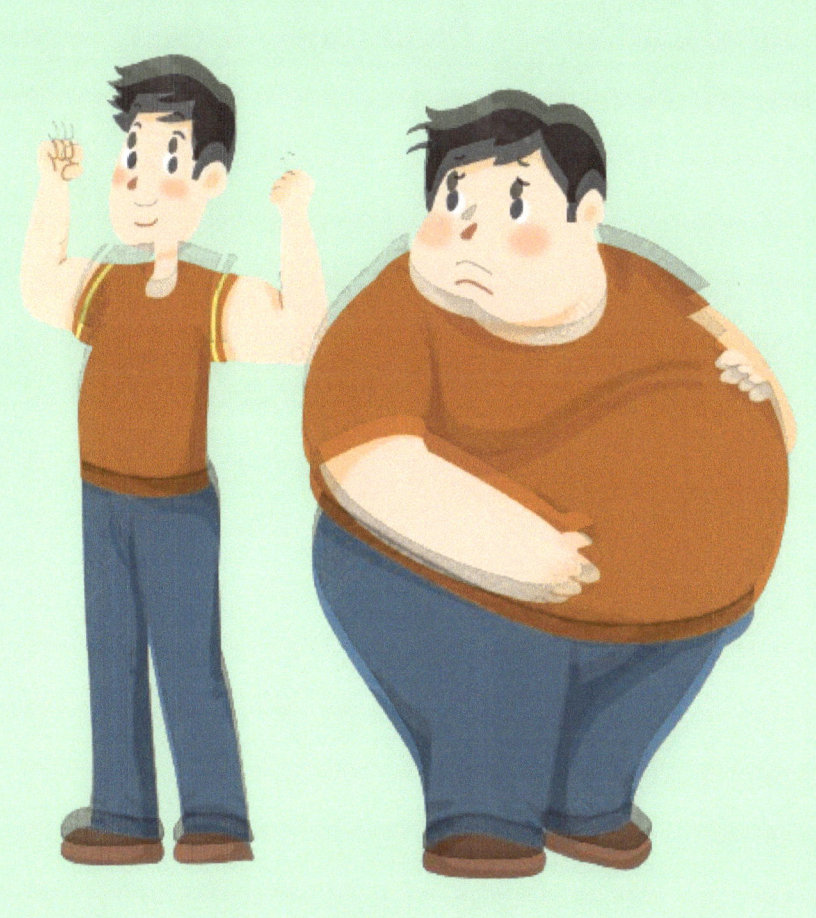

Health Implications

Obesity is associated with a range of health issues, including:

- **Cardiovascular Diseases:** Increased risk of heart disease and stroke.
- **Diabetes:** Particularly type 2 diabetes, due to insulin resistance.
- **Musculoskeletal Disorders:** Such as osteoarthritis.
- **Certain Cancers:** Including breast, colon, and endometrial cancer.
- **Respiratory Problems:** Like sleep apnea.

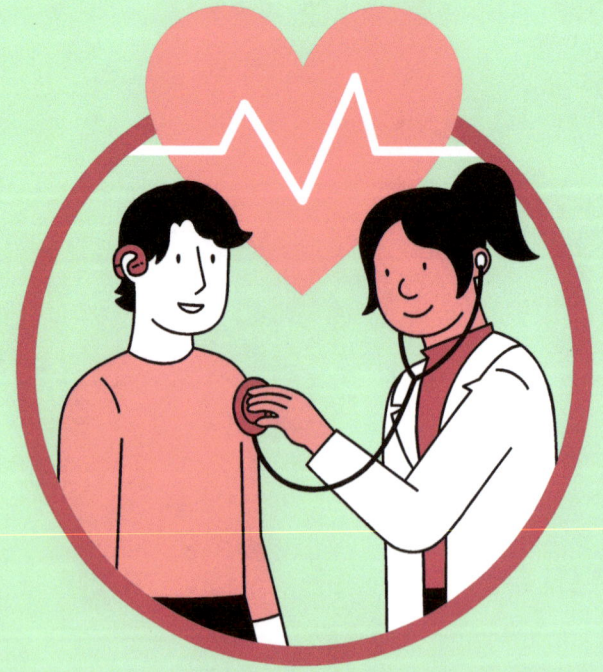

What are the Causes of Obesity?

Genetic Factors

Genetics can play a significant role in an individual's likelihood of becoming obese. Factors include:

- **Metabolism:** Genetic variations can affect how efficiently your body converts food into energy.
- **Fat Storage:** Genetics can influence how and where your body stores fat.
- **Appetite Regulation:** Hormonal imbalances, often influenced by genetics, can affect hunger and satiety.

Environmental Factors

The environment significantly influences obesity rates:

- **Diet:** High-calorie, low-nutrient foods are more accessible and affordable.
- **Physical Activity:** Sedentary lifestyles, driven by work and entertainment habits, reduce calorie expenditure.
- **Urbanization:** Infrastructure that discourages physical activity, like lack of sidewalks or parks.

Psychological Factors

Mental health can impact obesity through:
- Emotional Eating: Using food as a coping mechanism for stress, anxiety, or depression.
- Body Image Issues: Negative self-image can perpetuate unhealthy eating behaviors.

Socioeconomic Factors

Socioeconomic status affects access to:
- Healthy Foods: Limited access to fresh, nutritious food in some communities.
- Healthcare: Inadequate access to medical advice and treatment for weight management.
- Education: Lack of knowledge about nutrition and physical activity.

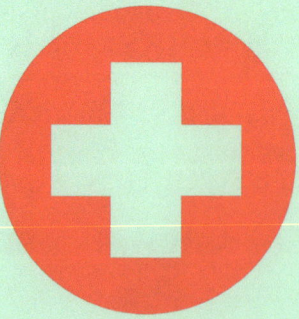

How to Handle Obesity

MEDICAL INTERVENTIONS

Medications

Prescription medications can help reduce appetite or increase feelings of fullness, but they are typically used in conjunction with lifestyle changes.

Surgery

Bariatric surgery, such as gastric bypass or sleeve gastrectomy, may be recommended for severe obesity when other interventions have failed.

LIFESTYLE CHANGES

Diet

Adopting a balanced diet rich in fruits, vegetables, lean proteins, and whole grains is crucial. Key strategies include:

- Portion Control: Reducing portion sizes to avoid overeating.
- Nutrient-Dense Foods: Prioritizing foods high in vitamins, minerals, and fiber

Physical Activity

Regular exercise is essential for weight management and overall health. Recommendations include:

- Aerobic Exercises: Activities like walking, running, or swimming.
- Strength Training: Building muscle mass to increase metabolism.

Behavioral Therapy

Psychological support can help address emotional and behavioral aspects of eating. Techniques include:

- Cognitive Behavioral Therapy (CBT): Changing negative thought patterns and behaviors.
- Support Groups: Sharing experiences and strategies with others facing similar challenges.

PREVENTIVE MEASURES

Public Health Initiatives

Policies and programs aimed at reducing obesity rates, such as:

- Nutrition Education: Providing information about healthy eating.

- **Physical Activity Promotion:** Creating environments that encourage active living.

Personal Habits

Adopting and maintaining healthy habits to prevent obesity, such as:

- **Regular Monitoring:** Keeping track of weight and health metrics.
- **Consistent Routines:** Establishing regular meal and exercise schedules.

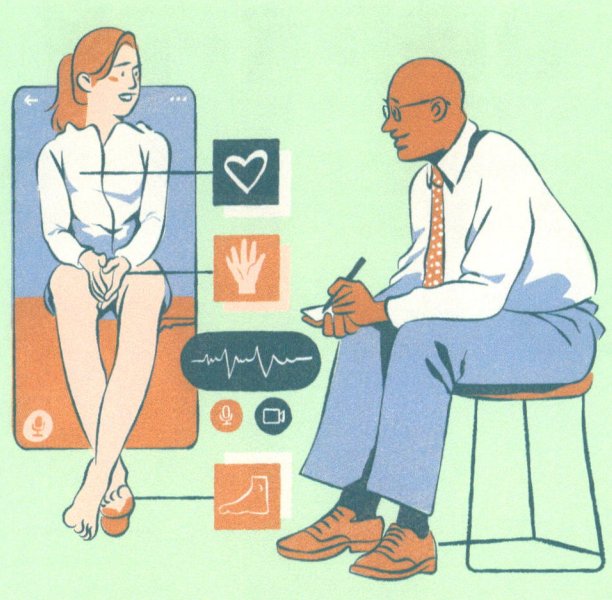

THE DANGERS OF OBESITY

Introduction to the Risks of Obesity

Obesity is more than a cosmetic concern; it is a serious medical condition that can have profound impacts on an individual's overall health and well-being. Understanding the dangers associated with obesity is crucial for recognizing the importance of addressing and managing this condition. This chapter explores the numerous health risks and complications linked to obesity, highlighting the need for proactive measures to combat it.

CARDIOVASCULAR HEALTH

Heart Disease

Obesity significantly increases the risk of heart disease, one of the leading causes of death worldwide. Excess body fat, particularly around the abdomen, contributes to:

- Hypertension (High Blood Pressure): Extra weight requires more blood to supply oxygen and nutrients to the body, leading to increased pressure on artery walls.
- High Cholesterol Levels: Obesity often leads to higher levels of LDL (bad) cholesterol and lower levels of HDL (good) cholesterol, promoting the buildup of fatty deposits in arteries.

- **Atherosclerosis:** The accumulation of fatty deposits (plaque) in the arteries can restrict blood flow, increasing the risk of heart attacks and strokes.

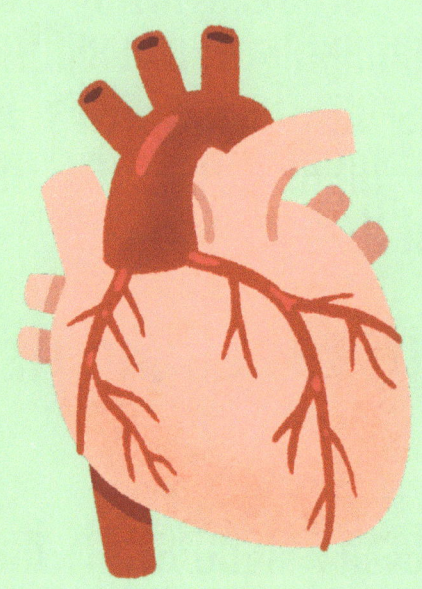

Stroke

Obesity is a significant risk factor for strokes due to its association with hypertension, high cholesterol, and diabetes. These conditions can lead to blockages or ruptures in the blood vessels supplying the brain, resulting in a stroke.

Metabolic and Endocrine Disorders

Type 2 Diabetes

Obesity is the leading cause of type 2 diabetes. Excess fat, particularly visceral fat around the abdomen, interferes with the body's ability to use insulin effectively, leading to insulin resistance and high blood sugar levels. Over time, this can result in:

- **Complications:** Kidney disease, nerve damage, vision problems, and an increased risk of heart disease.

Metabolic Syndrome

Metabolic syndrome is a cluster of conditions that occur together, increasing the risk of heart disease, stroke, and diabetes. It includes:

- **Abdominal Obesity:** Excess fat around the waist.
- **High Blood Pressure:** Elevated pressure on artery walls.
- **High Blood Sugar Levels:** Increased glucose levels due to insulin resistance.
- **Abnormal Cholesterol Levels:** Elevated triglycerides and reduced HDL cholesterol.

Respiratory Issues

Sleep Apnea

Obesity is a major risk factor for obstructive sleep apnea (OSA), a condition where the airway becomes blocked during sleep, causing repeated interruptions in breathing. This leads to:

- Poor Sleep Quality: Resulting in daytime fatigue, difficulty concentrating, and increased risk of accidents.
- Cardiovascular Problems: Increased risk of hypertension, heart disease, and stroke due to the strain on the cardiovascular system from repeated oxygen deprivation.

Asthma

Obesity can exacerbate asthma symptoms and increase the severity and frequency of asthma attacks. The excess weight can put additional pressure on the lungs, making it harder to breathe.

Musculoskeletal Issues

Osteoarthritis

Obesity places additional stress on weight-bearing joints, such as the knees, hips, and lower back. This can lead to the breakdown of cartilage and the development of osteoarthritis, causing:

- Chronic Pain: Persistent joint pain and stiffness.
- Reduced Mobility: Difficulty in performing daily activities and decreased quality of life.

Lower Back Pain

Excess weight, particularly in the abdominal area, can cause additional strain on the lower back, leading to chronic pain and discomfort.

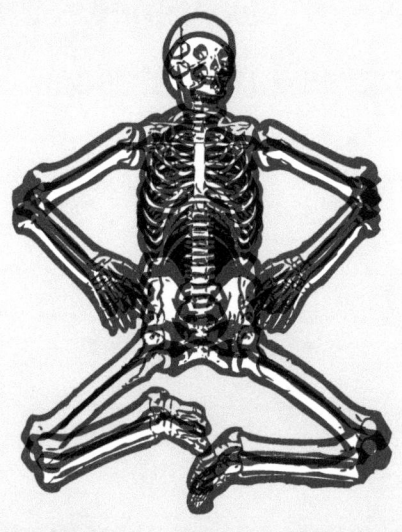

Cancer

Increased Cancer Risk

Obesity is linked to an increased risk of several types of cancer, including:

- Breast Cancer: Particularly in postmenopausal women.
- Colorectal Cancer: Excess fat can cause changes in the digestive system that increase cancer risk.
- Endometrial Cancer: Higher risk due to increased estrogen levels from excess fat tissue.
- Kidney Cancer: Obesity can affect kidney function and increase cancer risk.

Mechanisms

Obesity-related inflammation, hormonal imbalances, and insulin resistance can contribute to the development and progression of cancer.

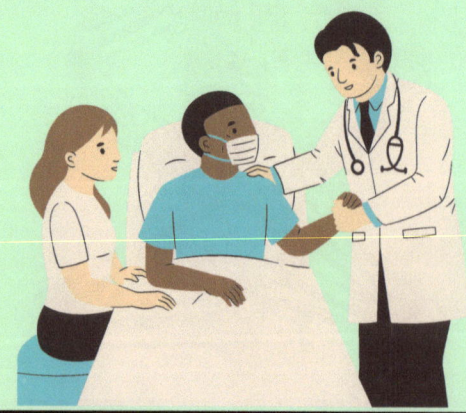

Mental Health

Depression and Anxiety

Obesity can have a profound impact on mental health, contributing to conditions such as:

- Depression: Stigma, discrimination, and low self-esteem associated with obesity can lead to depression.
- Anxiety: Concerns about health, appearance, and social interactions can cause increased anxiety.

Social Isolation

Obesity can lead to social isolation due to mobility limitations, low self-esteem, and societal stigma, further exacerbating mental health issues.

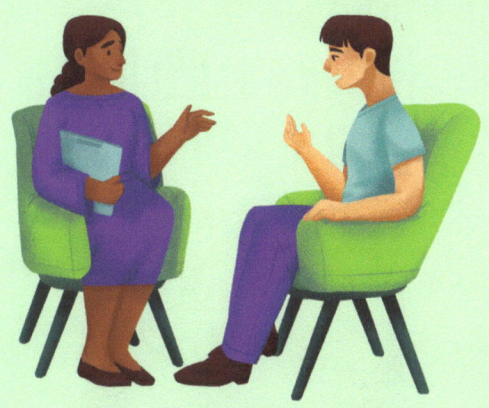

Reproductive and Sexual Health

Infertility

Obesity can impact fertility in both men and women. In women, excess weight can lead to hormonal imbalances, irregular menstrual cycles, and polycystic ovary syndrome (PCOS). In men, obesity can affect sperm quality and testosterone levels.

Complications During Pregnancy

Obesity during pregnancy increases the risk of complications such as:

- Gestational Diabetes: High blood sugar levels during pregnancy.
- Preeclampsia: High blood pressure and potential damage to other organs.
- Preterm Birth: Increased likelihood of delivering the baby before 37 weeks of gestation.

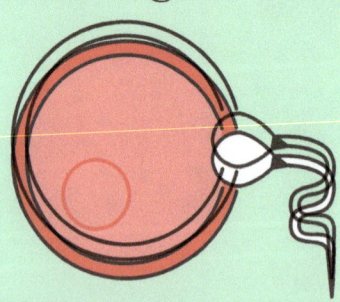

Understanding the dangers of obesity underscores the importance of addressing this condition through lifestyle changes, medical interventions, and supportive therapies. By recognizing the profound impact of obesity on physical and mental health, individuals can take proactive steps to reduce their risk and improve their overall well-being. The journey to a healthier life may be challenging, but the benefits of achieving and maintaining a healthy weight are invaluable, leading to a longer, more fulfilling life.

DIET AND OBESITY: A COMPREHENSIVE GUIDE

What is Diet?

Definition

A diet refers to the sum of food and drink that a person regularly consumes. It encompasses the choice of foods, the frequency and timing of meals, and the portion sizes. Diets can be tailored to meet specific health, cultural, or personal goals.

Types of Diets

There are various types of diets, including but not limited to:

- Balanced Diet: Incorporates a variety of food groups to ensure all essential nutrients are consumed.
- Weight Loss Diets: Focus on reducing calorie intake to promote weight loss.
- Medical Diets: Designed to manage specific health conditions, like diabetes or hypertension.
- Cultural/Traditional Diets: Reflect the culinary traditions and practices of a particular region or community.

How Diet Helps Recover from Obesity

Role of Diet in Weight Management

A well-planned diet plays a crucial role in managing and reducing obesity. It helps by:

- **Creating a Caloric Deficit:** Consuming fewer calories than the body needs forces it to use stored fat for energy.
- **Providing Essential Nutrients:** Ensures the body receives vitamins, minerals, and other nutrients necessary for overall health.
- **Regulating Metabolism:** Balanced meals can help maintain a steady metabolic rate.

Key Dietary Strategies

To effectively manage obesity through diet, consider the following strategies:

- **Portion Control:** Eating smaller portions to reduce overall calorie intake.
- **Nutrient-Dense Foods:** Prioritizing foods rich in nutrients but low in calories, such as vegetables, fruits, lean proteins, and whole grains.
- **Reducing Processed Foods:** Limiting foods high in added sugars, unhealthy fats, and empty calories.

• Hydration: Drinking plenty of water to support metabolism and reduce hunger.

Understanding Calories

What are Calories?

Calories are units of energy that measure the amount of energy food provides. The body uses this energy to perform essential functions such as breathing, circulation, and physical activity.

Caloric Needs

The number of calories a person needs varies based on several factors, including age, gender, weight, height, and activity level. To lose weight, one must consume fewer calories than their body expends.

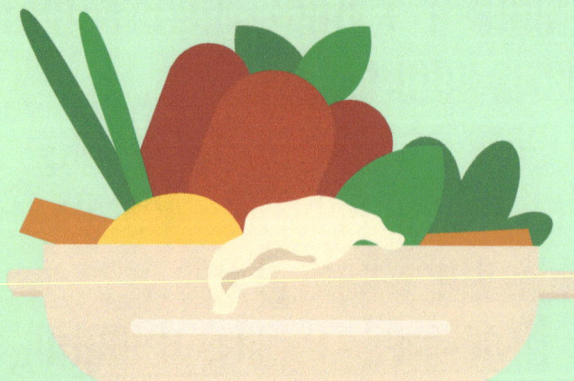

Calculating Caloric Intake for Weight Loss

To calculate caloric intake for weight loss:

Determine Basal Metabolic Rate (BMR):

The number of calories required to maintain basic bodily functions at rest.

Calculate Total Daily Energy Expenditure (TDEE):

The total number of calories burned per day, including physical activity.

Create a Caloric Deficit:

Aim to consume 500-1000 calories less than the TDEE for a safe weight loss of 0.5-1 kg per week.

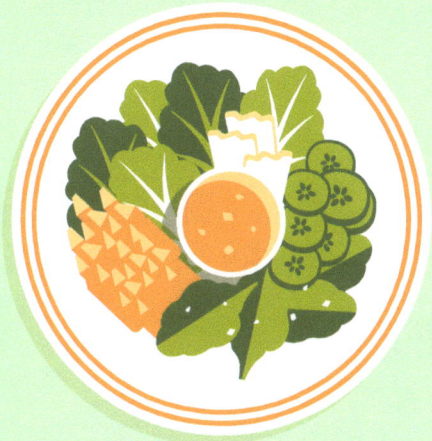

Sample Diet Plan with South Indian Foods (Calorie Calculation)

South Indian Diet Plan

Here's a sample South Indian diet plan designed to promote weight loss, with calorie calculations:

Breakfast
- Idli with Sambar: 2 idlis (120 calories) + 1 cup sambar (100 calories)
- Total Calories: 220

Mid-Morning Snack
- Fruit Salad: 1 cup mixed fruits (100 calories)
- Total Calories: 100

Lunch
- Brown Rice with Vegetable Curry: 1 cup brown rice (216 calories) + 1 cup vegetable curry (150 calories)
- Curd: 1/2 cup (55 calories)
- Total Calories: 421

Afternoon Snack
- Buttermilk: 1 glass (50 calories)
- Total Calories: 50

Dinner
- Ragi Dosa with Chutney: 2 ragi dosas (200 calories) + 2 tablespoons coconut chutney (100 calories)
- Total Calories: 300

Evening Snack
- Sprout Salad: 1 cup (150 calories)
- Total Calories: 150

Total Daily Calories: 1241

Nutritional Balance
This diet plan ensures a balance of carbohydrates, proteins, and fats while keeping the calorie count within a range conducive to weight loss. It also includes ample fiber from vegetables and whole grains, promoting satiety and digestive health.

Understanding diet and its critical role in managing obesity is essential for achieving and maintaining a healthy weight. By focusing on balanced, nutrient-dense foods and maintaining a caloric deficit, individuals can effectively reduce obesity and improve overall health. Adopting a diet plan that suits cultural preferences, such as the sample South Indian diet, can make the process enjoyable and sustainable.

NATUROPATHY AND YOGA: HOLISTIC APPROACHES TO MANAGING OBESITY

Introduction to Naturopathy and Yoga

What is Naturopathy?

Naturopathy is a holistic approach to health and wellness that emphasizes the body's inherent ability to heal itself. It integrates traditional natural therapies with modern medical science to promote overall well-being. Key principles of naturopathy include:

- Prevention and Treatment: Focus on preventing illness and treating the root cause of disease rather than just symptoms.
- Holistic Care: Considering the physical, mental, emotional, and spiritual aspects of health.
- Natural Therapies: Utilizing natural remedies, such as herbal medicine, nutrition, hydrotherapy, and lifestyle counseling.

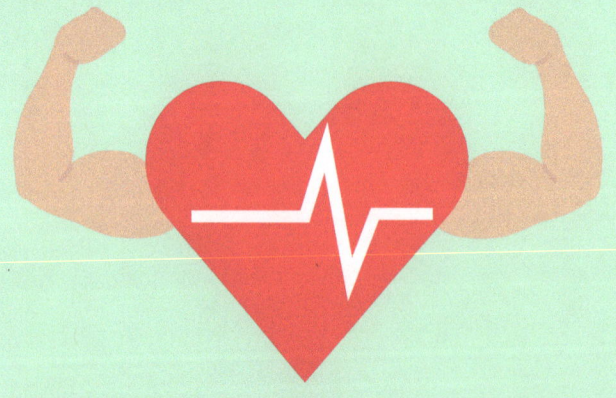

What is Yoga?

Yoga is an ancient practice that combines physical postures, breathing exercises, meditation, and ethical principles to promote physical, mental, and spiritual health. It has been practiced for thousands of years and offers numerous benefits, including:

- **Physical Fitness:** Improves strength, flexibility, and balance.
- **Mental Clarity:** Enhances focus, concentration, and mental calmness.
- **Emotional Stability:** Reduces stress, anxiety, and depression.
- **Spiritual Growth:** Encourages self-awareness and inner peace.

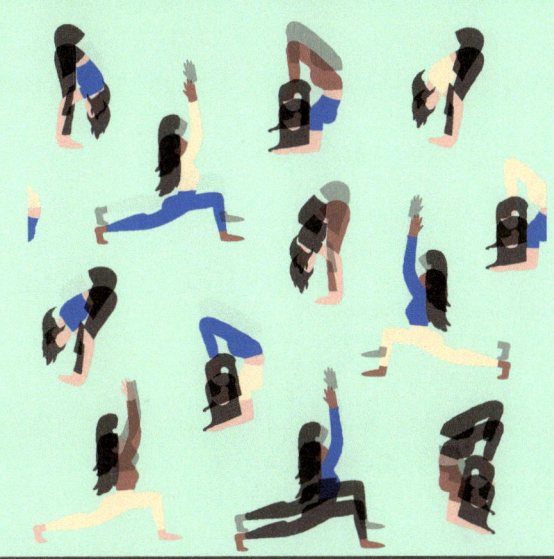

Naturopathy Treatment for Obesity

KEY PRINCIPLES OF NATUROPATHY IN OBESITY MANAGEMENT

Detoxification

Detoxification helps eliminate toxins from the body, which can improve metabolic function and aid weight loss. Methods include:

- Fasting: Short-term fasting or juice cleanses to reset the digestive system.
- Hydrotherapy: Using water-based treatments like baths, saunas, and enemas to cleanse the body.

Nutrition

A balanced, natural diet is crucial for managing obesity. Naturopathy emphasizes:

- Whole Foods: Consuming unprocessed, organic foods.
- Plant-Based Diet: Prioritizing fruits, vegetables, legumes, nuts, and seeds.
- Hydration: Drinking plenty of water to support metabolism and detoxification.

Herbal Medicine

Natural herbs can aid weight loss by boosting metabolism, reducing appetite, and enhancing digestion. Commonly used herbs include:

- Green Tea: Increases metabolic rate and fat oxidation.
- Garcinia Cambogia: Suppresses appetite and inhibits fat production.
- Dandelion: Acts as a diuretic and supports liver function.

Lifestyle Counseling

Naturopathy includes lifestyle modifications to promote weight loss, such as:

- Regular Physical Activity: Incorporating daily exercise routines.
- Stress Management: Techniques like meditation, deep breathing, and mindfulness.
- Sleep Hygiene: Ensuring adequate and quality sleep for optimal health.

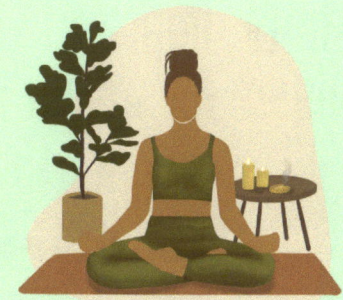

Yoga for Obesity Management

Yoga Postures (Asanas)

Certain yoga postures are particularly effective in promoting weight loss and improving overall fitness. These include:

- Sun Salutations (Surya Namaskar): A series of 12 poses that improve cardiovascular health and flexibility.
- Warrior Pose (Virabhadrasana): Strengthens the legs, arms, and core while enhancing stamina.
- Boat Pose (Navasana): Engages the abdominal muscles, promoting core strength and stability.
- Bridge Pose (Setu Bandhasana): Opens the chest and shoulders, strengthens the back, and stimulates the thyroid gland.

Breathing Exercises (Pranayama)

Pranayama involves controlling the breath to improve physical and mental health. Effective techniques for weight loss include:

- Kapalabhati (Skull Shining Breath): A vigorous breathing exercise that boosts metabolism and detoxifies the body.

- **Anulom Vilom (Alternate Nostril Breathing):** Balances the body's energy and reduces stress.
- **Bhastrika (Bellows Breath):** Increases oxygen supply, improves digestion, and energizes the body.

Meditation and Mindfulness

Meditation and mindfulness practices help manage emotional eating and reduce stress, which can contribute to obesity. Techniques include:

- **Mindful Eating:** Paying attention to the eating experience, savoring each bite, and recognizing hunger and fullness cues.
- **Guided Meditation:** Using meditation scripts or recordings to promote relaxation and mental clarity.
- **Yoga Nidra:** A form of guided relaxation that reduces stress and enhances body awareness.

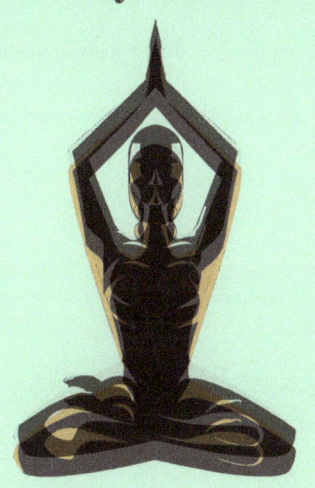

IMPORTANCE OF NATUROPATHY AND YOGA IN REDUCING OBESITY

Holistic Benefits

Naturopathy and yoga offer a holistic approach to obesity management, addressing physical, mental, and emotional aspects of health. Key benefits include:

- **Sustainable Weight Loss:** Encourages long-term lifestyle changes rather than quick fixes.
- **Improved Metabolic Health:** Enhances metabolic function and reduces risk factors associated with obesity, such as diabetes and cardiovascular diseases.
- **Enhanced Mental Well-Being:** Reduces stress, anxiety, and depression, which can contribute to overeating and weight gain.
- **Increased Physical Fitness:** Improves strength, flexibility, and endurance, making physical activity more enjoyable and effective.

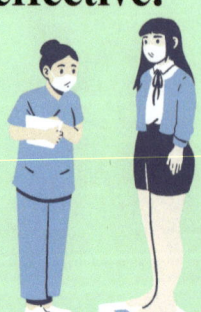

Integrative Approach

Combining naturopathy and yoga with conventional medical treatments can provide a comprehensive approach to obesity management. This integrative approach can:

- **Complement Medical Interventions:** Enhance the effectiveness of medical treatments and reduce side effects.
- **Promote Self-Care:** Empower individuals to take an active role in their health and well-being.
- **Encourage Mindful Living:** Foster a deeper connection between mind and body, promoting overall wellness.

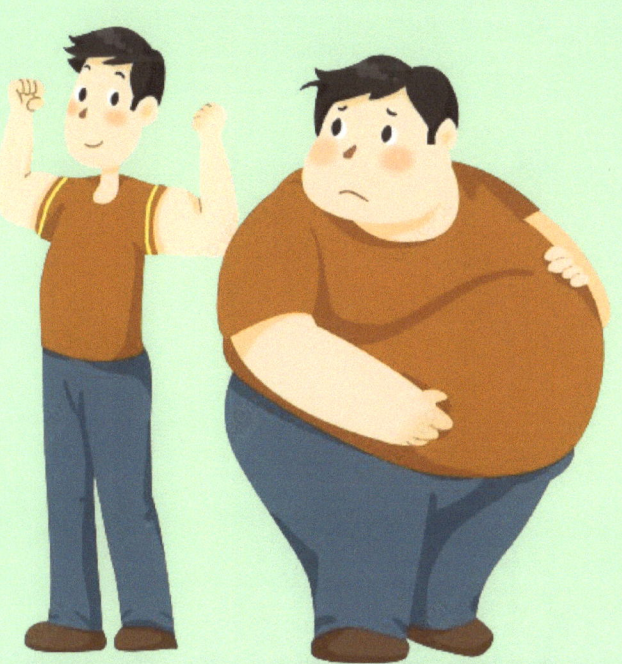

Naturopathy and yoga offer powerful tools for managing obesity through natural, holistic methods. By focusing on detoxification, nutrition, herbal medicine, and lifestyle modifications, naturopathy addresses the root causes of obesity. Meanwhile, yoga provides physical, mental, and emotional benefits that support sustainable weight loss and overall well-being. Integrating these practices into daily life can lead to lasting health improvements and a more balanced, fulfilling life.

MEDICATIONS FOR OBESITY: UNDERSTANDING AND MANAGING PHARMACOLOGICAL INTERVENTIONS

Introduction to Medications for Obesity

Overview

Medications for obesity, also known as weight-loss drugs or anti-obesity medications, are prescribed to aid in weight reduction for individuals who are obese or have weight-related health issues. These medications are typically used in conjunction with lifestyle modifications such as diet and exercise.

When Are Medications Recommended?

Weight-loss medications are generally recommended for individuals who:

- Have a Body Mass Index (BMI) of 30 or higher (obesity).
- Have a BMI of 27 or higher with obesity-related health conditions, such as diabetes, hypertension, or sleep apnea.
- Have not achieved adequate weight loss through diet and exercise alone.

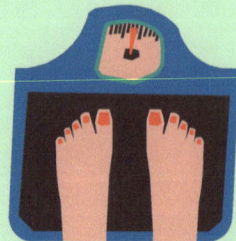

How Weight-Loss Medications Work

Mechanisms of Action

Weight-loss medications work through various mechanisms to help reduce body weight. The main mechanisms include:

Appetite Suppression

Some medications work by decreasing appetite or increasing feelings of fullness. This is typically achieved through the modulation of brain neurotransmitters.

- Example: Phentermine acts as an appetite suppressant by stimulating the release of norepinephrine, which helps reduce hunger.

Fat Absorption Inhibition

Certain medications prevent the absorption of fat from the diet, reducing overall calorie intake.

- Example: Orlistat inhibits the action of lipase, an enzyme needed to break down dietary fats, thus preventing fat absorption in the intestines.

Metabolism Enhancement

A few medications increase the body's metabolic rate, leading to higher energy expenditure:

- Example: Liraglutide, a GLP-1 receptor agonist, helps regulate appetite and increases the rate at which calories are burned.

Combination Medications

Some drugs combine different mechanisms to enhance weight-loss effects:

- Example: Phentermine-topiramate combines an appetite suppressant with an anticonvulsant that helps with weight loss.

Commonly Prescribed Weight-Loss Medications

PHENTERMINE

- Mechanism: Appetite suppressant.
- Side Effects: Increased heart rate, elevated blood pressure, insomnia, dizziness.

ORLISTAT

- Mechanism: Inhibits fat absorption.
- Side Effects: Gastrointestinal issues like oily stools, flatulence, and frequent bowel movements.

Liraglutide (Saxenda)

- Mechanism: GLP-1 receptor agonist; appetite suppression; increased metabolism.
- Side Effects: Nausea; diarrhea; constipation; low blood sugar.

Naltrexone-Bupropion (Contrave)

- Mechanism: Appetite suppression; increased energy expenditure.
- Side Effects: Nausea; constipation; headache; insomnia.

Phentermine-Topiramate (Qsymia)

- Mechanism: Appetite suppression; anticonvulsant.
- Side Effects: Tingling of hands and feet; dizziness; altered taste; insomnia.

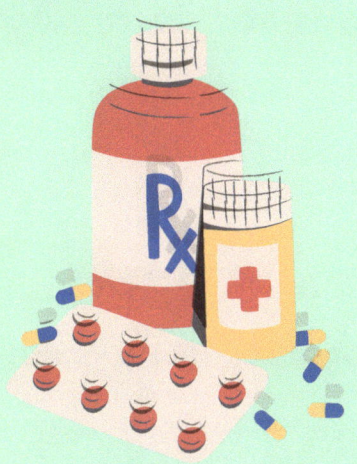

Side Effects and Risks of Weight-Loss Medications

Common Side Effects

While weight-loss medications can be effective, they may also cause side effects, such as:

- Gastrointestinal Issues: Nausea, diarrhea, constipation, and other digestive disturbances.
- Cardiovascular Effects: Increased heart rate, elevated blood pressure, and palpitations.
- Neurological Effects: Insomnia, dizziness, headache, and mood changes.

Serious Risks

In rare cases, weight-loss medications can lead to more serious health risks, including:

- Cardiovascular Events: Increased risk of heart attack or stroke.
- Psychiatric Issues: Depression, anxiety, and suicidal thoughts.
- Nutritional Deficiencies: Inhibition of fat absorption can lead to deficiencies in fat-soluble vitamins (A, D, E, K).

Obesity and Drug-Induced Weight Gain

MEDICATIONS THAT MAY CAUSE WEIGHT GAIN

Certain medications can contribute to weight gain as a side effect. These include:

ANTIDEPRESSANTS

- **Examples: Tricyclic antidepressants (TCAs), selective serotonin reuptake inhibitors (SSRIs) like paroxetine, and monoamine oxidase inhibitors (MAOIs).**
- Mechanism: Alterations in metabolism, appetite, and energy expenditure.

ANTIPSYCHOTICS

- Examples: Olanzapine, clozapine, risperidone.
- Mechanism: Changes in metabolism, increased appetite, and alterations in lipid and glucose metabolism.

ANTIDIABETIC MEDICATIONS

- Examples: Insulin, sulfonylureas.
- Mechanism: Promotion of fat storage and increased appetite.

CORTICOSTEROIDS

- Examples: Prednisone, hydrocortisone.
- Mechanism: Increased appetite, fluid retention, and redistribution of fat.

ANTIHISTAMINES

- Examples: Diphenhydramine, cetirizine.
- Mechanism: Increased appetite and sedation.

MANAGING DRUG-INDUCED WEIGHT GAIN

To manage weight gain caused by medications, consider the following strategies:

- Consult Healthcare Provider: Discuss potential alternatives or adjustments in medication.
- Lifestyle Modifications: Maintain a healthy diet and regular exercise routine.
- Monitoring and Support: Regularly monitor weight and seek support from healthcare professionals.

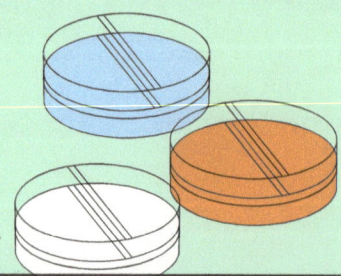

Medications for obesity can be an effective tool in managing weight when used appropriately and in conjunction with lifestyle changes. Understanding how these medications work, their potential side effects, and the impact of other drugs on weight is crucial for making informed decisions about obesity treatment. By working closely with healthcare providers, individuals can achieve better weight management and overall health outcomes.

YOUR PATH TO HEALTH: A PLANNER FOR ACHIEVING YOUR HEALTHY GOALS FROM OBESITY

Introduction

Embarking on a journey to overcome obesity and achieve a healthier lifestyle is a significant and commendable decision. This planner is designed to guide you step-by-step through the process of setting and achieving your health goals. It provides practical tools, strategies, and insights to help you stay motivated, track your progress, and make sustainable lifestyle changes. Remember, the journey to better health is a marathon, not a sprint. Take it one day at a time, and celebrate every small victory along the way.

SETTING YOUR HEALTH GOALS

Understanding Your Motivation

Before you start setting specific goals, take some time to reflect on your motivations for wanting to achieve a healthier weight. Ask yourself:

- Why do I want to lose weight?
- How will achieving a healthier weight improve my life?
- What are the long-term benefits I hope to gain?

SMART Goals

Set goals that are Specific, Measurable, Achievable, Relevant, and Time-bound (SMART). For example:

- Specific: "I want to lose 10 pounds in 3 months by following a balanced diet and exercising regularly."
- Measurable: Track your weight loss progress and other health indicators.
- Achievable: Set realistic goals based on your current lifestyle and capabilities.
- Relevant: Ensure your goals align with your overall health objectives.
- Time-bound: Set a timeline to achieve your goals.

Breaking Down Goals

Divide your main goal into smaller, manageable steps. For example:

- Week 1: Start incorporating more fruits and vegetables into your meals.
- Week 2: Begin a walking routine, aiming for 20 minutes a day.
- Week 3: Reduce sugary drinks and replace them with water or herbal tea.

NUTRITION PLANNING

Understanding Nutrition Basics

Learn about the fundamental principles of nutrition, including macronutrients (carbohydrates, proteins, and fats) and micronutrients (vitamins and minerals). Understand the importance of portion control and the role of different food groups in a balanced diet.

CREATING A MEAL PLAN

Develop a weekly meal plan that includes:

- Breakfast: Focus on high-fiber and protein-rich foods to start your day.
- Lunch: Include a balance of lean proteins, whole grains, and vegetables.
- Dinner: Opt for lighter meals with a good mix of protein, healthy fats, and greens.
- Snacks: Choose healthy options like fruits, nuts, and yogurt.

Sample Meal Plan: South Indian Diet

- **Breakfast:** Idli with sambar and coconut chutney (approximately 300 calories).
- **Mid-morning Snack:** A handful of almonds (approximately 100 calories).
- **Lunch:** Brown rice with dal, mixed vegetable curry, and a side salad (approximately 500 calories).
- **Afternoon Snack:** Fruit salad with a sprinkle of chia seeds (approximately 150 calories).
- **Dinner:** Ragi dosa with vegetable stew (approximately 350 calories).

Tracking Your Intake

Use a food diary or an app to log your meals and track your calorie intake. This helps you stay accountable and make informed choices.

EXERCISE AND PHYSICAL ACTIVITY

Finding the Right Exercise

Choose activities that you enjoy and that fit your lifestyle. Aim for a mix of cardio, strength training, and flexibility exercises.

Sample Exercise Plan

- Cardio: 30 minutes of brisk walking or cycling, 5 times a week.
- Strength Training: Bodyweight exercises like squats, push-ups, and lunges, 2-3 times a week.
- Flexibility: Yoga or stretching routines, 2-3 times a week.

Setting Exercise Goals

Set specific, achievable goals for your exercise routine. For example:

- Week 1: Walk for 15 minutes each day.
- Week 2: Increase walking time to 30 minutes.
- Week 3: Add a 10-minute strength training routine twice a week.

MONITORING PROGRESS

Regular Check-ins

Schedule regular check-ins to monitor your progress. This can include:

- Weekly weigh-ins.
- Monthly measurements (waist, hips, etc.).
- Tracking other health indicators (blood pressure, blood sugar levels, etc.).

Adjusting Your Plan

Based on your progress, make adjustments to your diet and exercise plan. Stay flexible and be willing to adapt as needed.

STAYING MOTIVATED

Finding Support

Seek support from family, friends, or a health coach. Join online communities or local support groups for encouragement and accountability.

Celebrating Milestones

Celebrate your achievements, no matter how small. Reward yourself with non-food-related treats, such as a new workout outfit, a massage, or a fun outing.

Overcoming Setbacks

Recognize that setbacks are a normal part of any journey. Learn from them and move forward without self-criticism. Stay focused on your long-term goals and remind yourself why you started.

INTEGRATING NATUROPATHY AND YOGA

Naturopathic Practices

Incorporate naturopathic practices such as:
- Hydrotherapy: Regular baths, saunas, or steam baths to support detoxification.
- Herbal Supplements: Consult with a naturopath for personalized herbal remedies to support weight loss and overall health.

Yoga for Weight Loss

Include yoga in your routine to enhance physical fitness, reduce stress, and improve mental clarity. Focus on poses that promote strength, flexibility, and relaxation.

Sample Yoga Routine

- **Sun Salutations (Surya Namaskar): A series of 12 poses to warm up and stretch your body.**
- **Warrior Pose (Virabhadrasana): Builds strength and stamina.**
- **Boat Pose (Navasana): Engages the core muscles.**
- **Bridge Pose (Setu Bandhasana): Strengthens the back and stimulates the thyroid gland.**

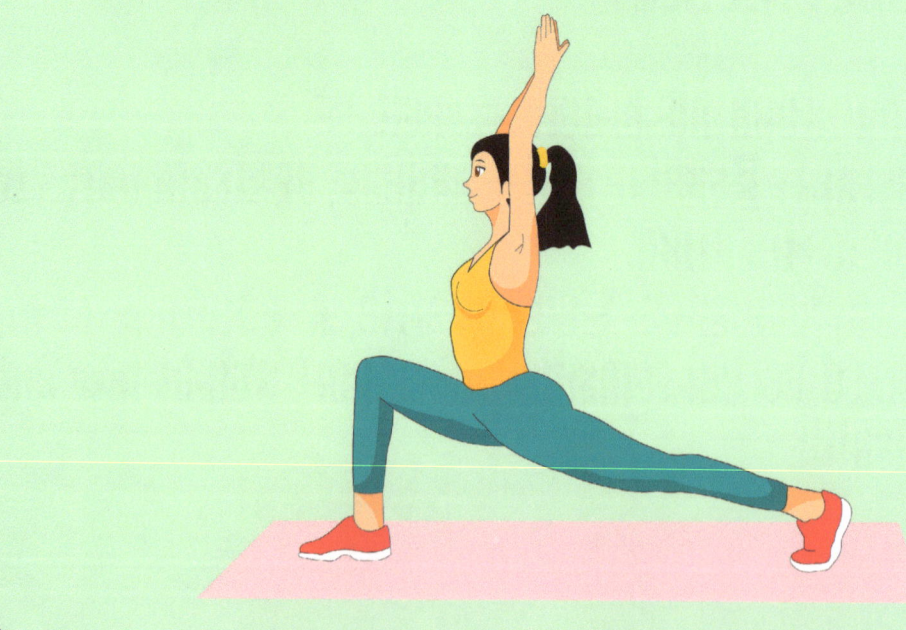

THE IMPORTANCE OF MENTAL AND EMOTIONAL HEALTH

Mindful Eating

Practice mindful eating by paying attention to your hunger and fullness cues, savoring each bite, and avoiding distractions while eating.

Stress Management

Incorporate stress management techniques such as meditation, deep breathing exercises, and progressive muscle relaxation to support mental and emotional well-being.

Building a Positive Mindset

Cultivate a positive mindset by setting realistic expectations, practicing self-compassion, and focusing on the progress you've made rather than perfection.

LONG-TERM SUCCESS

Maintaining Healthy Habits

Focus on maintaining the healthy habits you've developed, making them a permanent part of your lifestyle.

Regular Health Check-ups

Schedule regular check-ups with your healthcare provider to monitor your health and make any necessary adjustments to your plan.

Continuous Learning

Stay informed about the latest research and developments in health and wellness to keep improving your approach to maintaining a healthy weight.

Conclusion

Achieving your health goals and overcoming obesity is a journey that requires commitment, patience, and perseverance. By following this planner, you'll have a structured and supportive roadmap to guide you towards a healthier, happier life. Remember, every step you take brings you closer to your goals. Stay motivated, stay focused, and believe in your ability to make lasting, positive changes.

POSITIVE MESSAGES TO START USING THE PLANNER & OUR BOOK

WELCOME TO YOUR HEALTH JOURNEY

Dear Reader,

Congratulations on taking the first step toward a healthier, happier you! We are thrilled to accompany you on this transformative journey. This planner and book are designed to empower you with the knowledge, tools, and inspiration you need to achieve your health goals and overcome obesity. Every great journey begins with a single step, and today, you are taking that step. Here's why you should dive into this planner and make the most of your journey:

Embrace the Power of Change

"Every journey begins with a single step. Embrace that step today and pave the way for a healthier tomorrow."

Change can be daunting, but it also brings new opportunities for growth and improvement. By using this planner and book, you are making a powerful commitment to your health. Embrace each small change, knowing it leads to significant, positive transformations in your life.

Celebrate Your Progress

"Progress is progress, no matter how small. Celebrate each victory, for every step forward is a testament to your strength and determination."

Remember, every small victory counts. Whether it's choosing a healthier meal, taking a short walk, or practicing mindfulness, celebrate your progress. Each step you take brings you closer to your ultimate goal. Use this planner to track and celebrate your achievements, no matter how small they may seem.

Stay Motivated and Inspired

"Stay motivated, stay inspired, and let your journey to health be a testament to your resilience and commitment."

Staying motivated is key to achieving your health goals. Our book is filled with practical advice, uplifting stories, and evidence-based strategies to keep you inspired. Use the planner to set clear, achievable goals and stay on track. Let your journey be a source of inspiration for yourself and others.

EMPOWER YOURSELF WITH KNOWLEDGE

"Knowledge is power: Equip yourself with the right tools and information to make informed decisions and take control of your health."

Empower yourself with the knowledge contained in this book. Understand the science behind obesity, learn about nutrition, and discover effective exercise routines. Use the planner to apply this knowledge to your daily life. The more you know, the better equipped you'll be to make positive, lasting changes.

COMMIT TO A HEALTHIER YOU

"Commit to your health today. Your future self will thank you for the love and care you invest in yourself now."

Commitment is the foundation of success. By using this planner and book, you are committing to a healthier future. Your dedication today will pay off in the form of improved health, increased energy, and greater overall well-being. Trust in the process and stay committed to your goals.

SURROUND YOURSELF WITH SUPPORT

"You are not alone on this journey. Surround yourself with support and encouragement, and know that we are here with you every step of the way."

Support is crucial when embarking on a health journey. Share your goals with friends and family, join support groups, and lean on the resources provided in this book. Remember, we are here to support you every step of the way. Use the planner to connect with others and build a strong support network.

BELIEVE IN YOUR POTENTIAL

"Believe in yourself and your ability to change. You have the power to create a healthier, happier life."

Belief in yourself is a powerful motivator. Trust in your ability to make positive changes and overcome obstacles. This planner and book are tools to help you unlock your potential. Believe that you can achieve your health goals and let that belief drive your actions.

TAKE THE FIRST STEP TODAY

"The journey of a thousand miles begins with a single step. Take that step today, and let the journey to a healthier you begin."

There's no better time than now to start your journey. Open this book, begin using the planner, and take the first step toward a healthier you. Each page is designed to guide, motivate, and support you on your path to better health.

FINAL WORDS OF ENCOURAGEMENT

We believe in you and your ability to make lasting, positive changes. This planner and book are your companions on this journey, offering guidance, support, and inspiration. Embrace this opportunity, stay committed, and remember that every step you take brings you closer to your goals. Here's to your success and a healthier, happier you!

Mr. Jayaprathap Nagaraj,
Dr. Suvathi Vasan, and
Mr. Abinesh Kumar EPN

Calories Planning

Required Amount Of Calories____	Meal	Weight	Calories
Breakfast			
Lunch			
Dinner			
Snacks			

Calories Burned

Calories Need to Burn : _____

Calories Burned : _____

Notes

Workout Plan

Workouts	Counts

Required Amount Of Calories _____	Meal	Weight	Calories
Breakfast			
Lunch			
Dinner			
Snacks			

Calories Burned

Calories Need to Burn : _____

Calories Burned : _____

Notes

Workout Plan

Workouts	Counts

Calories Planning

Required Amount Of Calories	Meal	Weight	Calories
Breakfast			
Lunch			
Dinner			
Snacks			

Calories Burned

Calories Need to Burn : _____

Calories Burned : _____

Notes

Workout Plan

Workouts	Counts

Calories Planning

Required Amount Of Calories____	Meal	Weight	Calories
Breakfast			
Lunch			
Dinner			
Snacks			

Calories Burned

Calories Need to Burn : _____

Calories Burned : _____

Notes

Workout Plan

Workouts	Counts

Calories Planning

Required Amount Of Calories____	Meal	Weight	Calories
Breakfast			
Lunch			
Dinner			
Snacks			

Calories Burned

Calories Need to Burn : _____

Calories Burned : _____

Notes

Workout Plan

Workouts	Counts

Calories Planning

Required Amount Of Calories___	Meal	Weight	Calories
Breakfast			
Lunch			
Dinner			
Snacks			

Calories Burned

Calories Need to Burn : _____

Calories Burned : _____

Notes

Workout Plan

Workouts	Counts

Calories Planning

Required Amount Of Calories _____	Meal	Weight	Calories
Breakfast			
Lunch			
Dinner			
Snacks			

Calories Burned

Calories Need to Burn : _____

Calories Burned : _____

Notes

Workout Plan

Workouts	Counts

Calories Planning

Required Amount Of Calories____	Meal	Weight	Calories
Breakfast			
Lunch			
Dinner			
Snacks			

Calories Burned

Calories Need to Burn : _____

Calories Burned : _____

Notes

Workout Plan

Workouts	Counts

Calories Planning

Required Amount Of Calories____	Meal	Weight	Calories
Breakfast			
Lunch			
Dinner			
Snacks			

Calories Burned

Calories Need to Burn : _____

Calories Burned : _____

Notes

Workout Plan

Workouts	Counts

Calories Planning

Required Amount Of Calories	Meal	Weight	Calories
Breakfast			
Lunch			
Dinner			
Snacks			

Calories Burned

Calories Need to Burn : _____

Calories Burned : _____

Workout Plan

Workouts	Counts

Notes

Calories Planning

Required Amount Of Calories	Meal	Weight	Calories
Breakfast			
Lunch			
Dinner			
Snacks			

Calories Burned

Calories Need to Burn : _____

Calories Burned : _____

Notes

Workout Plan

Workouts	Counts

Calories Planning

Required Amount Of Calories____	Meal	Weight	Calories
Breakfast			
Lunch			
Dinner			
Snacks			

Calories Burned

Calories Need to Burn : _____

Calories Burned : _____

Notes

Workout Plan

Workouts	Counts

Calories Planning

Required Amount Of Calories____	Meal	Weight	Calories
Breakfast			
Lunch			
Dinner			
Snacks			

Calories Burned

Calories Need to Burn : _____

Calories Burned : _____

Notes

Workout Plan

Workouts	Counts

Calories Planning

Required Amount Of Calories	Meal	Weight	Calories
Breakfast			
Lunch			
Dinner			
Snacks			

Calories Burned

Calories Need to Burn : _____

Calories Burned : _____

Notes

Workout Plan

Workouts	Counts

Calories Planning

Required Amount Of Calories	Meal	Weight	Calories
Breakfast			
Lunch			
Dinner			
Snacks			

Calories Burned

Calories Need to Burn : _____

Calories Burned : _____

Notes

Workout Plan

Workouts	Counts

Calories Planning

Required Amount Of Calories____	Meal	Weight	Calories
Breakfast			
Lunch			
Dinner			
Snacks			

Calories Burned

Calories Need to Burn : _____

Calories Burned : _____

Notes

Workout Plan

Workouts	Counts

Calories Planning

Required Amount Of Calories___	Meal	Weight	Calories
Breakfast			
Lunch			
Dinner			
Snacks			

Calories Burned

Calories Need to Burn : _____

Calories Burned : _____

Notes

Workout Plan

Workouts	Counts

Calories Planning

Required Amount Of Calories_____	Meal	Weight	Calories
Breakfast			
Lunch			
Dinner			
Snacks			

Calories Burned

Calories Need to Burn : _____

Calories Burned : _____

Notes

Workout Plan

Workouts	Counts

Calories Planning

Required Amount Of Calories	Meal	Weight	Calories
Breakfast			
Lunch			
Dinner			
Snacks			

Calories Burned

Calories Need to Burn : _____

Calories Burned : _____

Notes

Workout Plan

Workouts	Counts

Calories Planning

Required Amount Of Calories____	Meal	Weight	Calories
Breakfast			
Lunch			
Dinner			
Snacks			

Calories Burned

Calories Need to Burn : _____

Calories Burned : _____

Notes

Workout Plan

Workouts	Counts

Calories Planning

Required Amount Of Calories___	Meal	Weight	Calories
Breakfast			
Lunch			
Dinner			
Snacks			

Calories Burned

Calories Need to Burn : _____

Calories Burned : _____

Notes

Workout Plan

Workouts	Counts

Calories Planning

Required Amount Of Calories _____	Meal	Weight	Calories
Breakfast			
Lunch			
Dinner			
Snacks			

Calories Burned

Calories Need to Burn : _____

Calories Burned : _____

Notes

Workout Plan

Workouts	Counts

Calories Planning

Required Amount Of Calories	Meal	Weight	Calories
Breakfast			
Lunch			
Dinner			
Snacks			

Calories Burned

Calories Need to Burn : _____

Calories Burned : _____

Notes

Workout Plan

Workouts	Counts

Calories Planning

Required Amount Of Calories____	Meal	Weight	Calories
Breakfast			
Lunch			
Dinner			
Snacks			

Calories Burned

Calories Need to Burn : _____

Calories Burned : _____

Notes

Workout Plan

Workouts	Counts

Calories Planning

Required Amount Of Calories____	Meal	Weight	Calories
Breakfast			
Lunch			
Dinner			
Snacks			

Calories Burned

Calories Need to Burn : _____

Calories Burned : _____

Notes

Workout Plan

Workouts	Counts

Calories Planning

Required Amount Of Calories	Meal	Weight	Calories
Breakfast			
Lunch			
Dinner			
Snacks			

Calories Burned

Calories Need to Burn : _____

Calories Burned : _____

Notes

Workout Plan

Workouts	Counts

Calories Planning

Required Amount Of Calories _____	Meal	Weight	Calories _____
Breakfast			_____
Lunch			_____
Dinner			_____
Snacks			_____

Calories Burned

Calories Need to Burn : _____

Calories Burned : _____

Notes

Workout Plan

Workouts	Counts
	_____
	_____
	_____
	_____
	_____
	_____

Calories Planning

Required Amount Of Calories____	Meal	Weight	Calories
Breakfast			
Lunch			
Dinner			
Snacks			

Calories Burned

Calories Need to Burn : _____

Calories Burned : _____

Notes

Workout Plan

Workouts	Counts

Calories Planning

Required Amount Of Calories____	Meal	Weight	Calories
Breakfast			
Lunch			
Dinner			
Snacks			

Calories Burned

Calories Need to Burn : _____

Calories Burned : _____

Notes

Workout Plan

Workouts	Counts

Calories Planning

Required Amount Of Calories _____	Meal	Weight	Calories
Breakfast			
Lunch			
Dinner			
Snacks			

Calories Burned

Calories Need to Burn : _____

Calories Burned : _____

Notes

Workout Plan

Workouts	Counts

Calories Planning

Required Amount Of Calories	Meal	Weight	Calories
Breakfast			
Lunch			
Dinner			
Snacks			

Calories Burned

Calories Need to Burn : _____

Calories Burned : _____

Workout Plan

Workouts	Counts

Notes